Sirtfood Diet Recipes

A Transforming Guide To The Sirtfood Diet Meal Plan Guide To Lose Weight, Eat Healthier, And Burn Fat By Activating Your Skinny Gene With Secret Recipes For A Healthy Diet Plan And Tasty Preparations

Serena Baxter

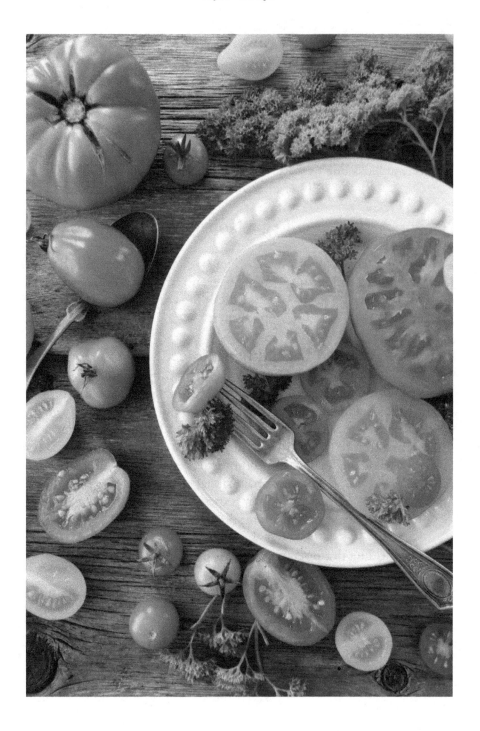

TABLE OF CONTENTS

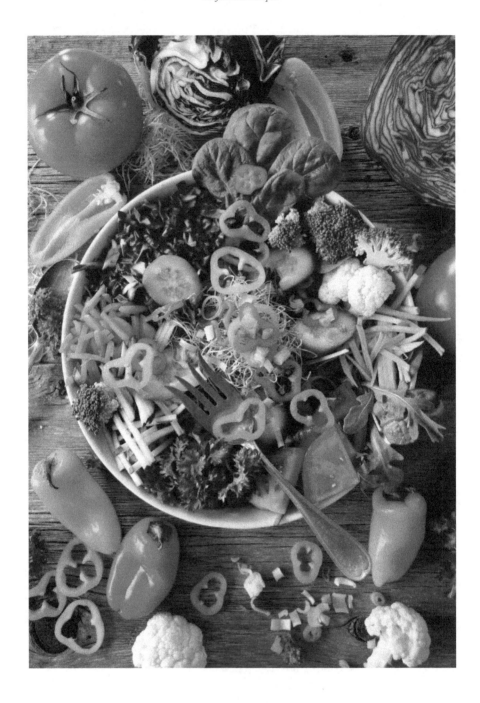

INTRODUCTION

The official Sirtfood Diet combines a short calorie restriction phase with a long-term commitment to nutrient-dense sirtuin-activating foods.

How you eat is your diet; restricting how you eat is dieting. Aside from the first week, Stage 1, the Sirtfood diet is not a traditional diet in that, instead of merely restricting calories, you focus on increasing nutrition and improving quality.

There are only 2 stages in the Sirtfood Diet, which take up 3 weeks of your life. Still, those 3 weeks are designed to set the stage for incorporating sirtfoods into your lifelong diet, eliminating your need to ever resort to dieting again.

The average American consumes many solid fats and sugars, refined grains, sodium, and saturated fat. They also under-consume vegetables, fruits, whole grains, and the nationally recommended intake of dairy and oils.

If this sounds like it matches your current eating patterns, don't be too hard on yourself, you're certainly not alone. And you've been practically brainwashed into adopting these poor nutrition habits. The number of fast-food restaurants continues to grow, as do your options for pre-made, packaged foods full of empty calories, and misleading promises. When you live on a diet of these foods devoid of all nutrition for too long, you find yourself getting sick and overweight. So, you turn to the industry that profits off of your poor health, the diet industry.

Sirtfood Diet is the newest approach to fast weight loss without extreme diet by stimulating the same 'skinny gene' mechanisms, typically just through fasting and exercise. Other foods varieties contain chemical substances known as polyphenols that stress our cells lightly, allowing genes to replicate the effects of fasting and exercise. The Sirtuin pathways, which affect metabolism, age, and mood, are guided by the food rich in polyphenols, like broccoli, dark chocolate, and red wine. However, a diet sufficient in these Sirtfoods starts to lose weight without sacrificing muscle while maintaining excellent health.

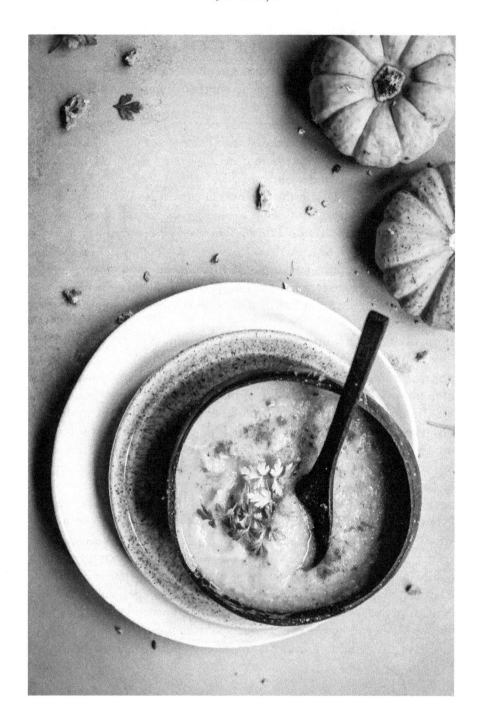

APPETIZER AND SNACK RECIPES

---

1. <u>Chocolate Chia Pudding with Almonds</u>

Preparation Time: 12 minutes

Cooking Time: 0 minute

Servings: 2

Ingredients:

- 4 tablespoons of chopped almonds

- 1 cup of water

- Sweetener

- ½ cup heavy cream

- 2 tablespoons of cocoa powder

- 6 tablespoons of chia seeds

- 2 tablespoons of MCT oil

Directions:

1. Add chia seeds, heavy cream, water, MCT oil, cocoa powder, and sweetener in a bowl.

2. Mix them. Allow sitting for 7-11 hours. After 11 hours, add almonds. Your dish is ready.

Nutrition: 288 Calories 28g Fat 8g Fiber

2. <u>Coconut Macadamia Chia Pudding</u>

Preparation Time: 12 minutes Cooking Time: 0 mins

Servings: 3

Ingredients:

- 4 tablespoons of macadamia nuts (chopped)

- 1 cup of water

- Sweetener

- ½ cup coconut cream

- 2 tablespoons of MCT oil

- 6 tablespoons of chia seeds

Directions:

1. Add chia seeds, coconut cream, water, MCT oil and sweetener in a bowl. Mix them.

2. Allow sitting for 7-11 hours.

3. After 11 hours add macadamia nuts.

Nutrition: 250 Calories 9g Fat 2g Protein

3. __Brownie Bites__

Preparation Time: 2 hours

Cooking Time: 0 minutes

Servings: 12

Ingredients:

- 2 ½ cups whole walnuts

- ¼ cup almonds

- 2 ½ cups Medjool0dates

- 1 cup cacao powder

- 1 teaspoon vanilla extract

- ¼ tsp. sea salt

Directions:

1. Blend all the ingredients using food processor.

2. Form into balls and situate on a baking sheet and freeze for 30 minutes.

Nutrition: 110 Calories 2.8g Fat 5g Protein

4. <u>Mascarpone Cheesecake</u>

Preparation Time: 12 minutes

Cooking Time: 23 minutes

Servings: 3

Ingredients:

Crust

- 1/2 cup slivered almonds

- 8 tsp. -- or 2/3 cup graham cracker crumbs

- 2 tbsp. sugar

- 1 tbsp. salted butter melted

Filling

- 1 (8-ounce) packages cream cheese, room temperature

- 1 (8-ounce) container mascarpone cheese, room temperature

- 3/4 cup sugar

- 1 tsp. fresh lemon juice (or imitation lemon-juice)

- 1 tsp. vanilla infusion

- 2 large eggs, room temperature

Directions:

1. For the crust: prep oven at 350 degrees. Get 9-inch diameter around the pan. Pulse almonds, cracker crumbs sugar in a food processor. Mix in butter

2. Press the almond mixture on the base of the prepared pan. Bake for 2 minutes. Lower temperature to 325 degrees F.

3. For your filling: with an electric mixer, scourge cream cheese, mascarpone cheese, and sugar. Pour in the lemon juice and vanilla. Add the eggs simultaneously until combined

4. Transfer cheese mixture on the crust from the pan. Position the pan into a big skillet then put enough hot water to the roasting pan. Bake for 1 hour Transfer

the cake to a stand 1 hour. Refrigerate before cheesecake is cold, at least eight hours.

5. Decorate the cake using melted chocolate

Nutrition: 5g Carbohydrates 25g Fat 5g Protein

5. <u>Chocolate Berry Blend</u>

Preparation Time: 32 minutes

Cooking Time: 0 minutes

Servings: 1

Ingredients:

- 2oz kale

- 2oz blueberries

- 2oz strawberries

- 1 banana

- 1 tablespoon 100% cocoa powder or cacao nibs

- 7 oz unsweetened soya milk

Directions:

1. Situate all of the ingredients into a blender with enough water to cover them and process until smooth.

Nutrition: 256 Calories 9g Fats6g Protein

BREAKFAST RECIPES

6. <u>Banana Pecan Muffins</u>

Preparation Time: 11 minutes

Cooking Time: 34 minutes

Serving: 6

Ingredients

- 3 Tbsp butter softened

- 4 ripe bananas

- 1 Tbsp honey

- 1/8 cup OJ

- 1 teaspoon cinnamon

- 2 cups all-purpose pasta

- 2 capsules a couple of pecans, sliced

- 1 Tbsp vanilla

Direction

1. Set oven to 350°F.

2. Grease bottom and sides of the muffin tin, and then dust with flour.

3. Dust the surfaces of the tin gently with flour then tap to eradicate any excess.

4. Peel and insert the batter to a mixing bowl and with a fork, mash the carrots; therefore, that you've got a combination of chunky and smooth, then put aside.

5. Insert the orange juice, melted butter, eggs, vanilla, and spices and stir to combine.

6. Roughly chop the pecans onto a chopping board, when using, then fold throughout the mix.

7. Spoon at the batter 3/4 full and bake in the oven for approximately 40 minutes, or until golden and cooked through.

Nutrition 167 Calories 9g Fat 12g Protein

7. <u>Banana and Blueberry Muffins - SRC</u>

Preparation Time: 13 minutes

Cooking Time: 42 minutes

Serving: 8

Ingredients

- 4 large ripe bananas, peeled and mashed

- 3/4 cup of sugar

- 1 egg, lightly crushed

- 1/2 cup of butter, melted

- 2 cups of blueberries

- 1 teaspoon baking powder

- 1 teaspoon baking soda

- 1/2 teaspoon salt

- 1 cup of coconut bread

- 1/2 cup of flour

- 1/2 cup applesauce

- dab of cinnamon

Direction

1. Situate mashed banana to a large mixing bowl.

2. Insert sugar & egg and mix well.

3. Add peanut butter and strawberries.

4. Sift all the dry ingredients together, then add the dry ingredients into the wet mix and mix together lightly.

5. Set into 12 greased muffin cups

6. Bake for 20-30min in 180C or 350 F.

Nutrition 161Calories 11g Fat 15g Protein

8. <u>Mushroom Scramble Egg</u>

Preparation Time: 7 minutes

Cooking Time: 13 minutes

Servings: 3

Ingredients

- Two eggs

- 1 teaspoon ground turmeric

- 1 teaspoon mild curry powder

- 20g kale, roughly chopped

- 1 teaspoon extra virgin olive oil

- ½ bird's eye chili, thinly sliced

- A handful of thinly sliced, button mushrooms

- 5g parsley, finely chopped

Directions

1. Mix the curry and turmeric powder, then add a little water until a light paste has been achieved.

2. Steam up the kale 2–3 minutes.

3. Over medium heat, cook oil in a frying pan and fry the chili and mushrooms for 2–3 minutes

4. Put the eggs and spice paste, and cook over medium heat, then add the kale and start cooking for another minute over medium heat. Add the parsley, then mix well and serve.

Nutrition: 185 Calories 27g fats 16g protein

9. <u>Sirtfood Eggs and Mushroom</u>

Preparation Time: 13 minutes

Cooking Time: 21 minutes

Servings: 1

Ingredients

- 2 medium eggs

- I teaspoon turmeric

- 1 ounce of kale, roughly chopped

- 1 teaspoon extra virgin olive oil

- 1/2 chili, thinly sliced

- 0.5 ounce of red onions

- Parsley, thinly chopped

- A handful of button mushrooms, thinly sliced

Direction

1. Smoke the kale for 2 minutes.

2. Dissolve turmeric powder with water.

3. Blend turmeric paste, parsley, and mix properly.

4. Warm up olive oil at medium heat then sauté onion, chili, and mushroom

5. Mix steamed kale to the mix in the frying pan.

6. Stir in egg mixture to the pan

7. Decrease heat and cook the egg.

Nutrition: 157 Calories 52g Protein 26g fats

10.Matcha Green Juice

Preparation Time: 8 minutes

Cooking time: 0 minutes

Servings: 2

Ingredients

- 5 ounces fresh kale

- 2 ounces fresh arugula

- ¼ cup fresh parsley

- ½ tsp. Matcha green tea

- 4 celery stalks

- 1 green apple, cored and chopped

- 1 (1-inch) piece fresh ginger, peeled

- 1 lemon, peeled

Direction

1. Incorporate the all ingredients then extract the juice as stated by the manufacturer's direction.

2. Fill into the glasses then serve.

Nutrition: 115 Calories 27g fat 11g protein

MAIN DISH RECIPES

11. Harvest Nut Roast

Preparation Time: 11 minutes

Cooking Time: 90 minutes

Serving: 4

Ingredients

- ½ cup celery, chopped
- 2 red onions, chopped
- ¾ cup walnuts
- ¾ cup pecan or sunflower meal
- 2 ½ cups soy milk
- 1 teaspoon dried basil
- 1 teaspoon dried lovage 3 cups breadcrumbs
- Salt and pepper to taste

Direction

1. Prep oven to 350 degrees F and lightly oil a loaf pan.

2. In a medium size skillet, sauté the chopped celery and onion in 3 teaspoons water until cooked.

3. In a large mixing bowl combine the celery and onion with walnuts, pecan or sunflower meal, soy milk, basil, lovage, breadcrumbs, and salt and pepper to taste; mix well.

4. Place mixture in the prepared loaf pan.

5. Bake for 60 to 90 minutes; until the loaf is cooked through.

Nutrition: 309 Calories 20g fat 45g Protein

12.Quick Spaghetti Sauce

Preparation Time: 9 minutes

Cooking Time: 30 minutes

Serving: 4

Ingredients

- 1 (29 ounce) can tomato sauce

- 1 cup mushrooms, chopped

- ½ cup chopped celery

- ¼ cup diced red onion

- ¼ cup Medjool dates, chopped

- ¼ cup walnuts, chopped 1 tomato, quartered

- 1 large orange, quartered

- 1 tablespoon garlic, minced

Directions

1. Using huge, heavy saucepan combine tomato sauce,

   mushrooms, celery, red onion, dates, walnuts, tomato,

orange and garlic. Cook on medium-high for 30 minutes.

2. Side with pasta or vegetable noodle alternative.

Nutrition: 317 Calories 30g fat 42g Protein

13.Spicy Ras-El-Hanout Dressing

Preparation Time: 13 minutes Cooking Time: 1 minute

Servings: 16

Ingredients:

- 125 ml Olive oil

- 1-piece Lemon (the juice)

- 2 teaspoons Honey

- 1 ½ teaspoons Ras el Hanout

- 1/2 pieces Red pepper

Directions:

1. Remove the seeds from the chili pepper.

2. Chop the chili pepper as finely as possible.

3. Place the pepper in a bowl with lemon juice, honey, and Ras-El-Hanout and whisk with a whisk.

4. Pour olive oil drop by drop while continuing to whisk.

Nutrition: 73 Calories 8g Fats 1g Carbohydrates

14.<u>Broccoli & Mushroom Chicken</u>

Preparation Time: 13 minutes

Cooking Time: 29 minutes

Servings: 5

Ingredients

- 3 tbsp. olive oil

- 1-pound chicken breast, cubed

- 1 medium onion

- 6 garlic cloves

- 2 cups fresh mushrooms

- 16 oz. broccoli florets

- ¼ cup water

Direction

1. Cook oil in a large wok over medium heat and fry chicken cubes for 4 minutes.

2. Situate chicken cubes onto a plate.

3. In the same wok, sauté onion for 4 minutes.

4. Cook mushrooms for 5 minutes.

5. Mix in the cooked chicken, broccoli, and water, and cook for 9 minutes, stirring occasionally.

6. Season well and remove from heat.

Nutrition: 196 Calories 11g Fat 21g Protein

15.Beef with Kale & Carrot

Preparation Time: 16 minutes

Cooking Time: 11 minutes

Servings: 4

Ingredients

- 2 tablespoons coconut oil

- 4 garlic cloves, minced

- 1-pound beef sirloin steak, cut into bite-sized pieces

- Ground black pepper, to taste

- 1½ cups carrots, peeled and cut into matchsticks

- 1½ cups fresh kale, tough ribs removed and chopped

- 3 tablespoons tamari

Direction

1. Melt the coconut oil in a wok over medium heat and sauté the garlic for about 1 minute.

2. Add the beef and black pepper and stir to combine.

3. Increase the heat to medium-high and cook for about 3–4 minutes or until browned from all sides.

4. Add the carrot, kale, and tamari, and cook for about 4–5 minutes.

5. Remove from the heat and serve hot.

Nutrition: 311 Calories 13.8g Fat 37g Protein

16.Lamb Chops with Kale

Preparation Time: 14 minutes

Cooking Time: 13 minutes

Servings: 4

Ingredients

- 1 garlic clove, minced

- 1 tablespoon fresh rosemary leaves, minced

- Salt and ground black pepper, to taste

- 4 lamb loin chops

- 4 cups fresh baby kale

Direction

1. Preheat the grill to high heat. Grease the grill grate.

2. In a bowl, add the garlic, rosemary, salt, and black pepper, and mix well.

3. Coat the lamb chops with the herb mixture generously.

4. Place the chops onto the hot side of grill and cook for about 2 minutes per side.

5. Now, move the chops onto the cooler side of the grill and cook for about 6–7 minutes.

6. Divide the kale onto serving plates and top each with 1 chop and serve.

Nutrition: 301 Calories 10g Fat 42g Protein

17.Chickpea with Swiss Chard

Preparation Time: 17 minutes

Cooking Time: 12 minutes

Servings: 4

Ingredients

- 2 tablespoon olive oil

- 2 garlic cloves, sliced thinly

- 1 large tomato, chopped finely

- 2 bunches fresh Swiss chard, trimmed

- 1 (18-ounce) can chickpeas, drained and rinsed

- Salt and ground black pepper, to taste

- ¼ cup water 1 tablespoon fresh lemon juice

- 2 tablespoons fresh parsley, chopped

Direction

1. Heat the oil in a big wok at medium heat and cook the garlic.

2. Add the tomato and cook for about 2–3 minutes, crushing with the back of spoon.

3. Cook remaining ingredients except lemon juice and parsley for 6 minutes.

4. Drizzle with the lemon juice and remove from the heat.

5. Serve hot with the garnishing of parsley.

Nutrition: 217 Calories 8.3g Fat 8.8g Protein

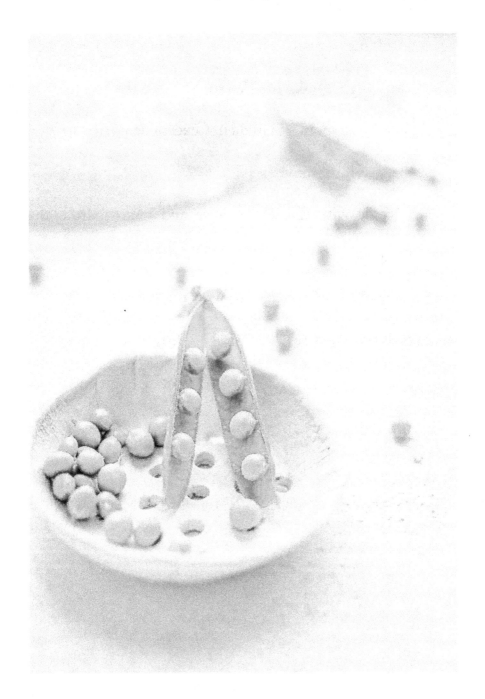

SIDES RECIPES

18.Apples and Cabbage Mix

Preparation Time: 7 minutes

Cooking Time: 0 minute

Servings: 4

Ingredients:

- 2 cored and cubed green apples

- 2 tbsps. balsamic vinegar

- ½ tsp. caraway seeds

- 2 tbsps. olive oil

- Black pepper

- 1 shredded red cabbage head

Directions:

1. Mix and toss cabbage with the apples and the other ingredients, then serve.

Nutrition: 165 Calories 7.4g Fat 2.6g Protein

19. Tofu Curry

Preparation Time: 18 minutes

Cooking Time: 31 minutes

Serving: 5

Ingredients:

- 1-liter water

- 1 tablespoon grapeseed oil

- 1 red onion – chopped

- 1 bird's eye chili

- 4 garlic cloves – chopped

- 1 teaspoon paprika

- ¼ teaspoon cayenne pepper

- ½ teaspoon turmeric – ground

- 7cm piece of ginger – grated

- 1 teaspoon salt

- 250 grams red lentils – dry

- 50 grams edamame beans – frozen

- 200 grams tofu – firm, cubed

- 1 lime - juiced

- 200 grams kale

- 2 tomatoes - chopped

Directions:

1. Put stove to low medium heat and put the oil in a pan. Add onions and cook for 5 minutes with occasional stirring. After the onions are cooked, add ginger, garlic, and chili.

2. Cook for 2 more minutes then add cumin, salt, cayenne, paprika, and turmeric. Stir the ingredients to combine with the onion mixture then add the lentils. As you are preparing this base for your dish, take a large cooking pot and pour 1 liter of water.

3. Boil water then add the boiling water to the pan to bring the ingredients to simmer for 10 minutes. Set

heat to low and allow the curry to cook for 20 to 30 minutes on low heat and until the consistency of the dish is porridge-like.

4. Add edamame beans, tofu, and tomatoes. Cook the curry for another 5 minutes after adding the three ingredients then add lime juice and kale. Cook until kale is softened. Serve warm and enjoy.

Nutrition: 342 Calories 5g Fat 28g Protein

20. <u>Veggie and Buckwheat Stir</u>

Preparation Time: 7 minutes Cooking Time: 32 minutes

Serving: 4

Ingredients:

- ½ cup buckwheat

- 3 tablespoons extra virgin olive oil

- 1 cup of water

- 1 medium carrot

- 1 medium red onion

- 1 red bell pepper -diced, deseeded

- 1 yellow bell pepper – diced, deseeded

- 10 grams parsley - chopped

Directions:

1. Take a heavy bottom pan and add buckwheat. Cook for 5 minutes on medium-low with frequent stirring and with no oil or water. Buckwheat can easily burn,

so make sure to stir while cooking for the first 5 minutes.

2. Cook 1 tablespoon of oil and stir in well. Mix and stir frequently until the oil is absorbed then add a cup of water.

3. Set heat to low, bring to a simmer, and cover with a lid. Cook for 20 minutes on low. Once you remove buckwheat from the heat don't open the lid but let it sit for another 20 minutes.

4. Pre-heat two tablespoons of oil in a skillet then add the onions, carrots, and peppers. Add some salt then stir to combine. Cook the veggies until softened.

5. Remove the lid from buckwheat then stir and add a sprinkle of salt. Add the sautéed veggies then stir to combine. Add parsley as a garnish and enjoy your meal.

Nutrition: 198 Calories 5g Fat 6g Protein

21.Sweet Pepper Mix

Preparation Time: 14 minutes Cooking Time: 0 minute

Serving: 3

Ingredients:

- 1/8 cup green bell pepper

- ¼ cup red bell pepper

- 1/8 cup yellow pepper

- 1/8 cup red onion

- ¼ cup rocket salad

- 1 tablespoon parsley – chopped

- ¼ lemon - juiced

Directions:

1. Dice the bell peppers, onion, and parsley and combine with rocket salad. Mix to combine in a salad bowl then dress with lemon juice.

Nutrition: 34 Calories 0.1g Fat 0.5g Protein

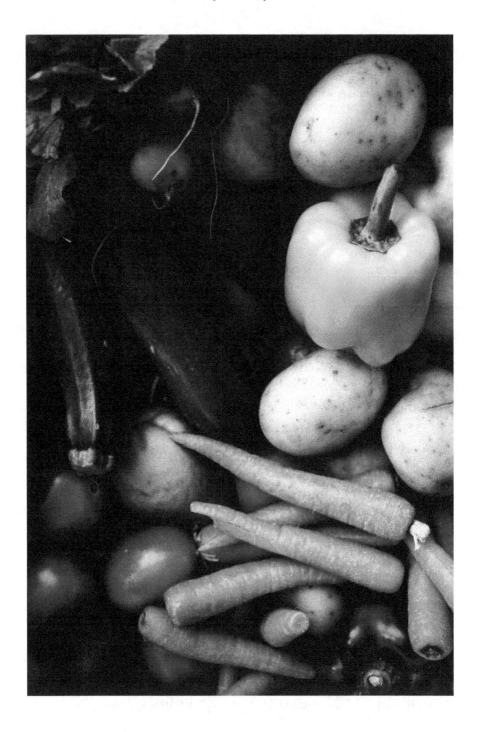

SEAFOOD RECIPES

22.   <u>Stir-Fried Greens, Sesame & Cod</u>

Preparation time: 16 minutes

Cooking Time: 11 minutes

Serving: 2

Ingredients:

- 20 g / 0.70 oz miso

- 1 tbsp mirin

- 1 tbsp extra virgin olive oil

- 200 g / 7 oz skinless cod fillet

- 20 g / 0.70 oz red onion, sliced

- 40 g / 1.4 oz celery, sliced

- 1 garlic clove, finely chopped

- 1 bird's eye chili, finely chopped

- 1 tsp finely chopped fresh ginger

- 60 g / 2.1 oz green beans

- 50 g / 1.7 oz kale, roughly chopped

- 1 tsp sesame seeds

- 5g / 1 tsp parsley, roughly chopped

- 1 tbsp tamari

- 30 g / 1 oz buckwheat

- 1 tsp ground turmeric

Direction

1. Blend miso, mirin, and 1 teaspoon of the oil. Brush all over the cod and marinate for 30 minutes. Set oven to 220°C/gas 7.

2. Bake the cod for 10 minutes.

3. Prep a frying pan with the remaining oil. Cook onion then mix celery, garlic, chili, ginger, green beans, and kale.

4. Cook the buckwheat following the packet's instructions for 3 minutes and sprinkle turmeric

5. Stir the sesame seeds, parsley, and tamari to the stir-

fry and serve with the greens and fish.

Nutrition: 321 Calories 19g Fat 9g Protein

23. <u>Turmeric Baked Salmon</u>

Preparation time: 23 minutes

Cooking time: 14 minutes

Serving: 2

Ingredients

- 125-150 g / 4.5- 5.5 oz Skinned Salmon

- 1 tsp Extra virgin olive oil

- 1 tsp ground turmeric

- ¼ Juice of a lemon

- For the spicy celery

- 1 tsp Extra virgin olive oil

- 40 g / 1.4 oz Red onion, finely chopped

- 60 g / 2 oz Tinned green lentils

- 1 Garlic clove, finely chopped

- 1 cm fresh ginger, finely chopped

- 1 Bird's eye chili, finely chopped

- 150 g / 1.7 oz Celery, cut into 2cm lengths

- 1 tsp Mild curry powder

- 130 g / 4.5 oz Tomato, cut into eight wedges

- 100 ml / ½ cup Chicken or vegetable stock

- 1 tbsp Chopped parsley

Direction

1. Heat oven to 200 ° C.

2. Start with hot celery. Pre-heat frying pan over medium-low heat, add the olive oil, then the onion, garlic, ginger, chili and celery. Fry for 2 minutes, then add the curry powder and cook for another minute.

3. Add the tomatoes, then the broth and lentils and simmer for 10 minutes.

4. Blend turmeric, oil, and lemon juice and rub the salmon. Situate on a baking sheet and cook for 9 minutes.

5. Combine parsley through the celery and serve with the salmon.

Nutrition: 328 Calories 21g Fat 13g Protein

VEGETABLE RECIPES

24. **Cottage Cheese and Vegetables**

Preparation Time: 9 minutes

Cooking Time: 13 minutes

Servings: 1

Ingredients:

- 6 cherry tomatoes

- ½ c. cottage cheese

- 2 tbsps. chopped scallion (green onion)

- 2 pimiento-stuffed green olives, sliced

- 1 tbsp. chopped fresh parsley (optional)

- Lettuce leaves

Directions:

1. Cut five tomatoes into quarters; reserve remaining tomato for garnish.

2. Mix all ingredients except lettuce and garnish.

3. Arrange salad plate with lettuce leaves, garnish with cheese mixture, and reserved cherry tomato.

Nutrition: 291 Calories 31g Protein 14g Fat

25. __Buckwheat Meatballs__

Preparation Time: 14 minutes

Cooking Time: 18 minutes

Serving: 4

Ingredients:

- 100 grams of buckwheat;

- 1 whole egg;

- a clove of garlic;

- a bunch of parsley;

- nutmeg;

- breadcrumbs;

- salt and pepper.

Directions

1. Wash the buckwheat and transfer it to a pot. Let it toast for a few seconds, after which add about

250/300 ml of cold water, sprinkle salt, and cook for 23 minutes.

2. Chop a clove of garlic and put it in a pan with a drizzle of oil, add the buckwheat well drained from the remaining cooking water and let it flavor together for a few minutes. Transfer everything into a bowl and let it cool.

3. When the wheat is warm, add the slightly beaten egg, nutmeg, finely chopped parsley, a pinch of pepper, and mix well.

4. Now form some balls with the help of a spoon and roll them in breadcrumbs. Compact the meatballs by squeezing them between the palms of your hands and, at the same time, flatten them slightly at the poles.

5. Grease a pan with oil and cook the meatballs on both sides until they are golden brown. Serve them hot

buckwheat meatballs accompanied by vegetables to taste.

Nutrition: 471 calories 16g fats 7g protein

26.   <u>Cabbage and Buckwheat Fritters</u>

Preparation Time: 11 minutes

Cooking Time: 4 minutes

Serving: 3

Ingredients:

- 20 g grated cheese

- 50 g cabbage tops

- 1 egg

- 1 tablespoon Flour 00

- 1/2 shallot

- Extra virgin olive oil

- Salt

Directions

1. Clean the cabbage and choose the florets. Finely cut the shallot and situate in the pressure cooker with 1 tablespoon of oil and the cabbage florets.

2. Brown gently, add the buckwheat and twice as much saltwater or vegetable broth. Close the pan and cook for 15 minutes from the start of the hiss.

3. Open the pot and let the mixture cool down. Add the egg and add enough flour to obtain a homogeneous mixture with a moderately firm consistency.

4. If necessary, add salt to taste. With floured hands, form round meatballs and then crush them slightly to flatten them.

5. Place them in a baking tray and brush them with a drizzle of oil. Bake them in the oven for 15 minutes at about 200 °C (392 °F)

Nutrition: 391 calories 12g fat 6g protein

27.   <u>**Buckwheat Salad with Artichokes**</u>

Preparation Time: 18 minutes

Cooking Time: 6 minutes

Serving: 4

Ingredients:

- 300 g buckwheat

- 200 g cherry tomatoes

- 5 artichokes 1 clove of garlic

- 1/2 cup large green olives

- fresh marjoram

- 5 tablespoons extra virgin olive oil

- salt 1 lemon

Directions

1. Using non-stick pan, toast the buckwheat grains, always stirring for 3 minutes, then boil salted water for 11 minutes. Drain and set aside.

2. Clean the artichokes: remove the outer leaves, trim them and remove the beard, cut them into segments, and throw them away as they are cleaned in water acidulated with lemon juice, so that they do not blacken.

3. In the meantime, brown the clove of garlic dressed lightly crushed in two tablespoons of oil.

4. When the artichokes are all hulled and cut, drain them and put them in the pan. Brown them without burning, then lower the heat and cook until they have softened a bit; they must remain al dente. Remove the garlic clove and sprinkle with a little fresh marjoram.

5. Put the buckwheat in the pan with the artichokes, stir well, and cook for a couple of minutes to make it taste good. Turn off and set aside.

6. Rinse and chop the cherry tomatoes in 2, leaving them a little in a colander to drain the vegetation water.

7. Slice olives in half and remove the stone.

8. Incorporate the cherry tomatoes and olives with buckwheat, add more marjoram leaves, stir and let them flavor well covered, over low heat.

Nutrition: 341 calories 21g fat 15g protein

28.   **Pasta with Rocket Salad and Linseed**

Preparation Time: 21 minutes

Cooking Time: 21 minutes

Serving: 4

Ingredients:

- 400 gr of whole meal pasta

- 1 bunch of washed and dried Rocket

- 1 tablespoon of peeled almonds

- 1 tablespoon Linseed

- 1/2 clove of Garlic

- 4 spoons of extra virgin olive oil

- 3 tablespoons of water (if necessary)

- A few drops of lemon juice Salt Pepper

Directions

1. First, wash the arugula and put it to dry on a kitchen

   cloth, then boil water and throw the dough;

2. In a mixer, add 1 tablespoon of linseed, 1 tablespoon of almonds, half a clove of garlic (without the sprout) and 4 tablespoons of oil;

3. Cut everything for a few minutes, if necessary, add a little water to make the pesto more fluid;

4. At this point add the rocket, a few drops of lemon juice, a pinch of salt and turn the mixer again for a few seconds, then add salt and pepper, and your pesto is ready;

5. Before draining the pasta, set aside some cooking water so that it can be used later, in case the pesto is too thick;

6. Once drained, put the pasta on the pot, season it with the pesto, and, if necessary, add a little cooking water previously-stored; continuing to stir for about a minute, and now your dish is ready to taste!

Nutrition: 401 calories 29g fat 17g protein

29.   <u>Sirt Yogurt</u>

Preparation Time: 7 minutes

Cooking Time: 0 minutes

Serving: 1

Ingredients

- 125g mixed berries

- 150g Greek yogurt

- 25g of chopped walnuts

- 10g of dark chocolate (85 percent cocoa) grated

Directions

1. Put your favorite berries in a bowl and pour yogurt on top. Sprinkle them with nuts and chocolate.

2. For a vegan alternative, you can replace Greek yogurt with soy or coconut milk.

Nutrition: 297 calories 27g fat 11g protein

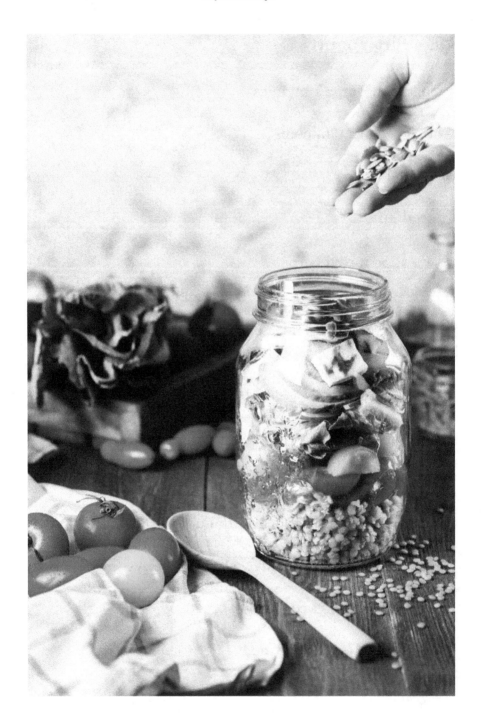

SOUP AND STEW RECIPES

30. <u>Cauliflower Kale Curry</u>

Preparation Time: 13 minutes

Cooking Time: 32 minutes

Serving: 4

Ingredients:

- 200 g buckwheat

- 2 tbsp ground turmeric

- 1 red onion, chopped

- 3 cloves of garlic, minced

- 2.5 cm piece of fresh ginger, chopped

- 1–2 chili peppers, chopped

- 1 tbsp coconut oil

- 1 tbsp mild curry powder

- 1 tbsp ground cumin

- 2 × 400 g cans of chopped tomatoes

- 300 ml vegetable broth

- 200 g kale, roughly chopped

- 300 g cauliflower, chopped

- 1 × 400 g can of butter beans, drained

- 2 tomatoes, cut into wedges

- 2 tbsp chopped coriander

Direction:

1. Cook the buckwheat following to the instructions on the package and add 1 tablespoon of turmeric to the water.

2. In the meantime, cook the onion, garlic, ginger and chili peppers in the coconut oil over medium heat for 2-3 minutes.

3. Add the seasonings, including the remaining tablespoon of turmeric and continue cooking over low to medium heat for 1–2 minutes.

4. Add the canned tomatoes and the broth and bring to a boil then simmer for 10 minutes.

5. Add the kale, cauliflower and butter beans and cook for 10 minutes.

6. Add the tomato wedges and coriander and cook for another minute.

7. Then serve them with the buckwheat.

Nutrition 17g Fat 8g Protein 270 Calories

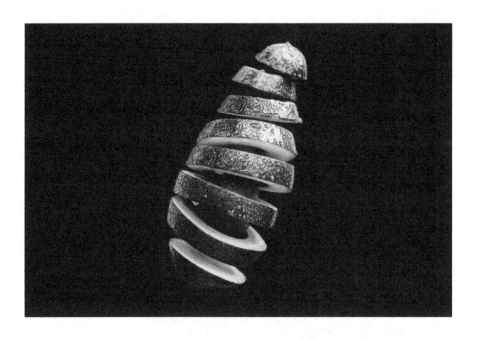

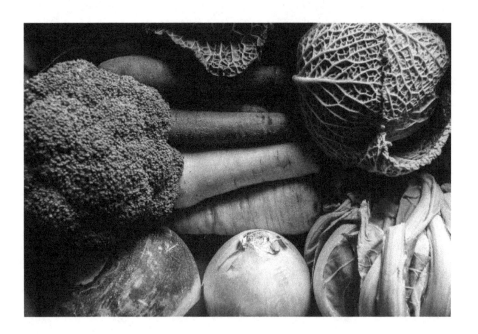

VEGETARIAN RECIPES

31.Potatoes with Onion Rings in Red Wine

Preparation Time: 11 minutes

Cooking Time: 32 minutes

Serving: 4

Ingredients:

- Diced potatoes, 3 cups

- Extra virgin olive oil, 1 tbsp

- Finely chopped parsley, ½ tbsp

- Red wine, 1 tbsp

- Vegetable stock, 150ml

- Tomato sauce, 1 tsp

- 1 sliced red onion

- Kale, sliced, 1 cup

- A pinch of salt

- A pinch of pepper

- 1 chopped bird's eye chili

Direction:

1. Boil the potatoes for up to five minutes and drain. Roast at 22o °C for 45 minutes. Add the parsley after taking the potatoes out of the oven.

2. Fry the onions for up to seven minutes in 1 tsp of olive oil and add kale and garlic. Add vegetable stock and let boil for up to two minutes. Serve alongside potatoes.

Nutrition: 341 calories 19g fats 8g protein

SALAD RECIPES

32. Avocado, Tomato, Arugula Salad

Preparation: 13 minutes Cooking: 0 minute Serving: 2

Ingredients

- 1 cup Orange tomatoes

- 1/2 cup chopped avocado

- 1/2 cup arugula radish

- 1 cup Red Tomatoes

Dressing:

- 1 tbsp. olive oil

- 1 tbsp. fresh lemon juice

- pinch of black pepper

- pinch of sea salt

Direction:

1. Mix all ingredients.

Nutrition: 119 Calories 5g Fat 10g Protein

33. <u>Chicken, Tomato, Arugula & Cucumber</u>

<u>Salad</u>

Preparation: 7 minutes Cooking: 0 minute Serving: 2

Ingredients

- 1 cup grilled chicken

- 1/2 cup chopped cucumber

- 1/2 cup chopped tomato

- 1 cup arugula

Dressing:

- 1 tbsp. olive oil or avocado oil

- 1 tbsp. fresh lemon juice

- pinch of black pepper

- pinch of sea salt

Direction:

1. Mix all ingredients.

Nutrition: 207 Calories 6g Fat 4g Protein

34.   Artichoke, Arugula & Lamb Salad

Preparation Time: 6 minutes

Cooking Time: 22 minutes

Serving: 2

Ingredients

- 1 cup sliced roasted lamb

- 1 cup roasted quartered artichoke hearts.

- 1/2 cup chopped red onion

- 1 cup Arugula

Dressing:

- 1 tbsp. olive oil or avocado oil

- 1 tbsp. fresh lemon juice

- pinch of black pepper

- pinch of sea salt

Direction:

1. Roast artichoke hearts for 20 minutes in the oven.

2. Mix all ingredients.

Nutrition: 207 Calories 11g Fat 7g Protein

35. <u>Smoked-Tender Salmon Sirt Salad</u>

Preparation Time: 24 minutes

Cooking Time: 0 minutes

Servings:4

Ingredients:

- 1 cup, or ¼ package if large of smoked salmon slices

- 1 avocado, pitted, sliced, and scooped out

- 10 walnuts, chopped

- 5 lovage or celery leaves), chopped

- 2 celery stalks, chopped or sliced thinly

- ½ small red onion, sliced thinly

- 1 Medjool pitted date, chopped

- 1 tbsp. capers

- 1 tbsp. extra virgin olive oil

- 1/4 of a lemon, juiced

- 5 sprigs of parsley, chopped

Directions:

1. Wash and dry salad makings and vegetables, top with salmon.

Nutrition: 214 Calories 2g Protein 9g Fat

36. Coronation Chicken Salad

Preparation Time: 28 minutes

Cooking time: 0 minutes

Servings: 1

Ingredients:

- 75 g Natural yoghurt

- Juice of 1/4 of a lemon

- 1 tsp Coriander, chopped

- 1 tsp Ground turmeric

- 1/2 tsp Mild curry powder

- 100 g Cooked chicken breast, cut into bite-sized pieces

- 6 Walnut halves, finely chopped

- 1 Medjool date, finely chopped

- 20 g Red onion, diced

- 1 Bird's eye chili

- 2-ounce Rocket, to serve

Direction

1. Blend the yoghurt, lemon juice, coriander and spices together in a bowl. Add all the remaining Ingredients and serve on a bed of the rocket.

Nutrition: 122 Calories 13g Fat 9g Protein

37.   <u>Salad Buckwheat Pasta</u>

Preparation: 26 minutes Cooking: 22 minutes Serving: 1

Ingredient

- 2 ounces of buckwheat pasta, cooked according to the directions for packaging

- Big pound of rye

- Tiny pound of basil leaves

- 8 Halved cherry tomatoes

- 1/2 Avocado 10 olives diced

- 1 Tablespoon of extra virgin olive oil

- 21/2 spoonful of pine nuts

Direction

1. Combine all the ingredients, except the pine nuts, gently and place them on a tray, then spread the nuts over the edges.

Nutrition: 322 Calories 17g Fat 8g Protein

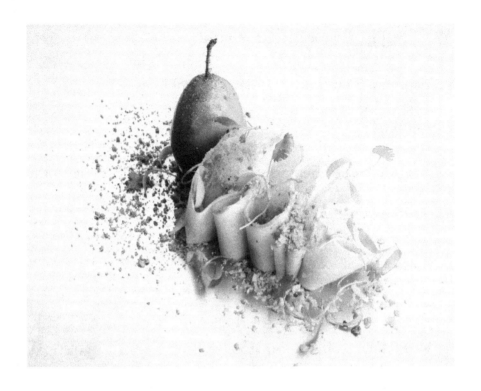

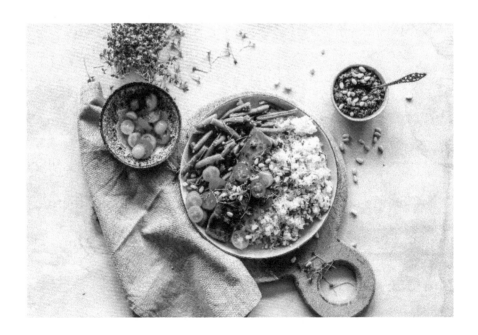

DESSERT RECIPES

38.   <u>Chocolate Orange Cheesecake</u>

Preparation Time: 18 minutes

Cooking Time: 1 hour

Serving: 10

Ingredients

- 800g (1¾ lb.) cream cheese

- 4 medium eggs

- 50g (2oz) 100% cocoa powder

- 2 teaspoons stevia sweetener powder (or to taste)

- 5 tablespoons freshly squeezed orange juice

Direction

1. Situate all of the ingredients into a bowl and combine them. Test the sweetness of the mixture and add extra stevia if necessary.

2. Transfer the mixture to a pie dish and bake at 170C/325F for one hour. Remove the cheesecake and allow it to cool. Serve chilled.

Nutrition: 400 Calories 27g Protein 22g Fat

39.   <u>**Strawberry Pretzel Salad**</u>

Preparation Time: 46 minutes

Cooking time: 11 minutes

Servings: 4

Ingredients:

Pretzel Crust

- 3 1/2 cups pretzels, squashed

- 1/4 cup sugar

- 1/2 cup unsalted spread, dissolved

Cream Cheese Filling

- 8 Oz cream cheddar, mellowed

- 1/2 cup sugar

- 8 Oz cool whip, or whipped cream (solidly whipped)

- Strawberry Jell-O Topping

- 1 lbs. new strawberries, hulled and cut

- 2 cups bubbling water

- 6 Oz strawberry jelly powder

Directions:

1. Preheat stove to 350°F. Put aside a 9x13 inch glass preparing dish. Spot pretzels in a Ziplock sack, seal and pound with a moving pin to smash daintily. In a medium bowl, mix together the liquefied margarine and sugar.

2. Include the squashed pretzels and blend to cover. Press the pretzel blend into the preparing dish, and afterward heat for 10 minutes. Expel from broiler. In a medium bowl, consolidate jelly powder with bubbling water.

3. Mix gradually for one moment until broke down and put in a safe spot. In a huge bowl, beat the cream cheddar and sugar until soft. Utilizing a huge spatula, crease in the cool whip until equitably mixed.

4. When the prepared pretzels are cool, spread the cream cheddar blend equitably on top until level over the dish. At that point, chill for at any rate 30 minutes. While chilling, you can wash, body and cut the strawberries.

5. Tenderly spot the cut strawberries onto the filling in a solitary layer. Include any residual strawberries top as a fractional second layer. When the Jell-O blend is room temperature, spill over the strawberries utilizing the rear of a spoon for even dispersion. Chill for in any event two hours. Serve and appreciate it!

Nutrition: 200 Calories 9g Carbohydrates 2g Fats

40. <u>Sheet Pan Apple Pie Bake</u>

Preparation Time: 22 minutes

Cooking Time: 16 minutes

Servings: 1

Ingredients:

- 8 flour tortillas, 8 inches

- 4 tbsp unsalted spread

- 8 Granny Smith apples, stripped, cored and cleaved

- 3/4 cup sugar, partitioned

- 3 tsp cinnamon, partitioned

- 1 tbsp lemon juice, new pressed

- Serving thoughts - discretionary

- whipped cream   frozen yogurt   caramel sauce

Directions:

1. Preheat stove to 400°F. Put aside a medium preparing sheet. On a medium preparing sheet, orchestrate 6

tortillas in a blossom petal design with a few creeps outside the dish and a few crawls of cover.

2. Spot a seventh tortilla in the center. Spot an enormous skillet on medium-high warmth. Include spread, slashed apples, 1/2 cup sugar and 2 tsp cinnamon. Sauté the apples for 8-10 minutes until they begin to relax, mixing normally with a wooden spoon.

3. Spoon apple blend from skillet over tortillas on prepared sheet. Spread out to make an even layer. Overlay the folds of tortilla outside the dish over the apples. Spot the eighth tortilla in the center to cover the hole.

4. Blend staying 1/4 cup sugar with 1 tsp cinnamon. Sprinkle equally over the tortillas. Spot another preparing dish on top to hold the tortillas set up and

heat for 20 minutes. Expel from the stove and permit to cool for 5-10 minutes.

5. Present with discretionary frozen yogurt, whipped cream and caramel sauce. Appreciate!

Nutrition: 250 Calories 2g Fats 4g Carbohydrates

CONCLUSION

Thanks for making it to the end of sirtfood diet cookbook. Sirtfood diet plan is a great plan that like all plans need to be implemented with a great deal of effort, discipline and determination. Sirtfood diet can help you lose weight if you fully implement it into your life and make it a habit.

As stated above this diet is not supposed to be a short-term plan but a long-term lifestyle goal. You cannot implement this diet and then revert to your normal eating habits. You need to adopt lifestyle changes. If you wish to lose weight and stay fit, then you need to do something about it.

It is suggested to eat sirtfood diet recipes every day. The future benefits of sirtfood diet will overcome any initial discomfort you might feel during the beginning phases of the diet. If you wish to make this diet successful, then you need to believe in it.

I hope you have enjoyed reading Sirtfood Diet Plan.

Good luck on your sirtfood journey!

CPSIA information can be obtained
at www.ICGtesting.com
Printed in the USA
BVHW062305140621
609528BV00011B/2022